AROMATHERAPY
Essential Oils
for Healing

Demetria Clark

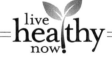

live
hea|thy
now!

HEALTHY LIVING PUBLICATIONS
Summertown, Tennessee

© 2015 Demetria Clark

Cover and interior design: Scattaregia Design

Healthy Living Publications,
a division of Book Publishing Company
PO Box 99
Summertown, TN 38483
888-260-8458
bookpubco.com

ISBN 978-1-57067-322-1

20 19 18 17 16 15   1 2 3 4 5 6 7 8 9

Library of Congress Cataloging-in-Publication Data

Clark, Demetria.
Aromatherapy essential oils for healing / Demetria Clark.
   pages cm
ISBN 978-1-57067-322-1 (pbk.) -- ISBN 978-1-57067-872-1 (e-book)
1. Aromatherapy. I. Title.
RM666.A68C53 2015
615.3'219--dc23
                2014049751

Printed on recycled paper

Book Publishing Company is a member of Green Press Initiative. We chose to print this title on paper with 100% post-consumer recycled content, processed without chlorine, which saved the following natural resources:

• 18 trees

• 563 pounds of solid waste

• 8,414 gallons of water

• 1,551 pounds of greenhouse gases

• 8 million BTUs of energy

For more information on Green Press Initiative, visit greenpressinitiative.org. Environmental impact estimates were made using the Environmental Defense Fund Paper Calculator. For more information, visit papercalculator.org.

CONTENTS

Aromatherapy for Body, Mind, and Spirit

Aromatherapy, simply defined, is the process of using scents for healing. It's a very easy and practical everyday therapy to use at home; in fact, many types of aromatherapy applications can be made at home (see page 31). Topical applications, which are applied directly to the skin, include body sprays, creams, compresses, liniments, and massage oils. Alternatively, scents can be diffused into the surrounding air or dispersed through steam and inhaled.

Aromatherapy has many uses and multiple potential benefits. It's effective cosmetically, for skin and hair care, or it can be used to target deeper issues, such as specific physical, emotional, and mental health concerns.

Aromatherapy works because the system involved in the sense of smell, the olfactory system, connects the nose with points in the brain that comprise the limbic system. Here lies the amygdala, hippocampus, and hypothalamus, parts of the brain that are concerned primarily with emotion and motivation. When stimulated by smell, the limbic system releases chemicals that affect the central nervous system, influencing physical, emotional, and mental health.

From our own individual experiences, we know that anything we smell in our natural environment can stimulate sometimes strong reactions. The powerful sense of smell can evoke attachments, feelings, and memories. For example, scent attracts people to potential mates and promotes a bond between a new baby and its parents. In fact, whether we're aware of it or not, the sense of smell activates our most primal emotions, including fear, love, and lust.

Each brain processes scent differently. For example, the scent of lavender typically makes people feel relaxed and at ease. However, for some people, lavender may smell unpleasant, or it may cause them to feel agitated or restless. It's important for anyone who uses aromatherapy, from a professional aromatherapist to someone who occasionally uses a diffuser at home, to be aware that scents don't elicit the same reactions in every aromatherapy user.

A Short History of Modern Aromatherapy

The term "aromatherapy" was coined in 1928 by chemist René-Maurice Gattefossé, who was inspired to study and write about essential oils after an explosion in his lab. His hand was badly burned, and he treated his wounds with lavender essential oil. When his burns healed remarkably quickly, he was inspired to investigate essential oils further.

Influenced by the work of Gattefossé, French physician Jean Valnet used essential oils as antiseptics while treating wounded soldiers during World War II. He continued his use and scientific study of essential oils, eventually publishing his classic text, *L'armathérapy*, in France in 1964. The English version, *The Practice of Aromatherapy*, is still available. Valnet's approach of matching the healing properties of a specific plant with the needs of the patient remains the backbone of modern aromatherapy. His work has inspired many well-known aromatherapists, including Micheline Arcier, Julia Lawless, Marguerite Mary, Shirley Price, and Robert Tisserand, and me.

Essential Oils

The scents used in aromatherapy are typically essential oils, or concentrated plant oils. Despite the name, essential oils are not all that oily because they're not true oils but rather the essence of plant components. Essential oils are found in the flowers, fruits, leaves, roots, seeds, and stems of plants. Most are clear, but some are amber, brown, orange, or yellow, depending on the color of the plant source.

There are different ways to extract an essential oil from a plant. The most common method is water distillation. Other essential oils are expressed, and some are extracted using ancient techniques. Following are some common extraction methods:

Distillation. The most popular method of obtaining essential oils is through steam distillation. Anyone who is familiar with how an old-fashioned moonshine still works knows the basics of distillation: water is heated to the boiling point, then the resulting steam passes through fresh plant material that has been placed above the boiling water. The steam pressure is carefully controlled. When the steam passes through the plant material, it causes the plant's cell walls to swell and break down. This allows the essential oil to be released as vapor. Then the essential oil vapor and water pass through a condenser that cools the steam and the oil into a liquid. Because essential oils don't dissolve in water, the two can be separated. Essential oils that are lighter than water rise to the top and are then siphoned off. Essential oils that are heavier than water sink to the bottom and can be collected.

Enfleurage. An ancient technique for extracting essential oils is enfleurage, which involves the application of odorless fats and oils to plants to absorb the plants' essential scent qualities. In the past, this process was typically used to extract the essential oils of highly scented, fatty flowers, such as honeysuckle and jasmine. This method is not commonly used in the making of modern essential oils.

Expression. Expression is a method that physically forces the essential oil from a plant. For example, components of a citrus plant may be pressed to obtain the essential oil. You can witness an example of expression simply by peeling an orange. When you bend the rind, the orange's essential oil sprays forth, creating a visible display (if you look closely) and coating your fingers with an enticing scent. Expression is also known as cold-pressing, and the resulting oils may be referred to as cold-pressed extractions.

Absolutes and Hydrosols

Essential oils aren't the only plant products used in aromatherapy. Two other ingredients used in aromatherapy are absolutes and hydrosols.

Absolute. Despite the fact that absolutes are often displayed and sold right beside essential oils, an absolute is not considered a pure essential oil but instead falls into a classification of its own. An absolute is obtained through chemical solvent extraction. The solvent used is alcohol, and the alcohol is removed with vacuum extraction. The most common absolutes are jasmine, rose, and sandalwood.

Hydrosol. When an essential oil is produced by distillation, the aromatic water that remains is the hydrosol. While essential oils should be diluted for topical use, hydrosols are more dilute and considered safe for topical use without dilution. Hydrosols are commonly sold wherever essential oils are sold and can be safely added to all kinds of hair- and skin-care products, such as creams, facial toners, liniments, and lotions.

Aromatherapy Applications

Essential oils can be used in bath salts, body sprays, liniments, massage oils, salves, and many more wonderful topical applications. They also can be healing when diffused into the air or inhaled. To learn how to make essential oil therapies at home, see the methods on page 28 and the recipes on pages 31 to 46.

Topical Applications

Because they can be very strong, with few exceptions, essential oils should be diluted before being applied to the skin. Dilution is the best way to prevent reactions or sensitivities. Typically, essential oils are diluted with a carrier oil, such as a nut, seed, or vegetable oil (see page 27). When it's safe to apply an essential oil directly to the skin, it is said that the oil can be applied "neat," or without dilution.

Body Sprays

Body sprays are used to tone the skin, and they can be quite cooling and refreshing. In addition, their effects can go much deeper. The can effectively lift moods, energize, and ease anxiety or stress. Body sprays are very easy to make and use.

Creams and Lotions

Any cream or lotion that you already have can be enhanced with essential oils. Ideally, mix essential oils with an unscented cream or lotion, using a brand that works well for you. Most people prefer to apply a light cream on the body and a thick cream on the face (especially overnight) or on dry skin anywhere on the body.

Compresses

A compress is made by soaking a piece of clean cloth (such as linen, cotton, or gauze) in hot or cold water mixed with one or more essential oils. For example, one of my favorite compresses for sports injuries contains lavender and Roman chamomile essential oils.

Liniments

A liniment is a combination of an essential oil and food-grade alcohol, such as vodka, or witch hazel. Liniments are rubbed into the skin to provide relief from arthritis, sore muscles, strains, and inflammations of the ligaments, muscles, and tendons. Do not use rubbing alcohol to make a liniment since it can irritate the skin, eyes, and mucous membranes.

Massage Oils

Massage oils are made by combining a carrier oil and essential oils or infused oils. After mixing, all massage oils should be transferred to a clean, dry glass bottle, sealed, and stored in a clean, dry place.

Salves

A salve has a firmer texture than a cream or lotion and is made by combining essential oils and beeswax, coconut oil, or another firm base. Like creams and lotions, salves are applied directly to the skin to treat physical ailments. They also can be helpful in treating emotional issues.

Inhaling Essential Oils

Perhaps one of the easiest forms of aromatherapy is inhalation. This involves breathing in, or inhaling, an essential oil to obtain the oil's healing benefits. The essential oil travels through the nose and mouth to the lungs, making inhalation an especially great form of therapy for head colds and sinus ailments. Simply removing the bottle cap and inhaling an essential oil can be therapeutic, particularly to aid breathing.

When you want a portable remedy, add a few drops of essential oil to a small bottle that contains a few large grains of rock salt. For example, use eucalyptus, peppermint, or rosemary essential oils to clear the nasal passages. If you anticipate stressful events, use clary sage, grapefruit, lavender, mandarin, or sweet orange essential oils to keep calm.

Another quick remedy to relieve congestion or enhance respiratory function is to inhale essential oils in steam. For example, the "over-the-bowl" method involves boiling water, pouring it into a bowl, and adding 3 to 7 drops of essential oil. Lean over the bowl, place a towel over your head and the bowl (forming a makeshift tent to contain the steam), and inhale for about 5 minutes. To avoid burns, be careful not to get your face too close to the water or the steam and avoid knocking over the bowl.

Diffusing Essential Oils

When an essential oil is diffused, it's dispersed into the surrounding air with a device called a diffuser. Diffusing is considered one of the most effective ways to deliver the healing benefits of essential oils in aromatherapy. See the box on page 11 for a list of the positive effects that can be obtained through diffusion.

Note that a humidifier is *not* an essential oil diffuser, although many people use essential oils in humidifiers at the risk of damaging either its plastic or electronic parts. Rather, an essential oil diffuser is a device designed specifically to break down the oil particles and disperse them in the air. Using a diffuser is ideal but not necessary; simply putting an essential oil on a cotton ball or in a sachet will allow the scent and benefits to spread over time.

When using an essential oil diffuser, be sure to use only pure essential oils. If you use anything artificial, you will be at risk of breathing in chemicals and synthetics. Feel free to try different diffusers; you may find that you prefer a certain type for a specific application. Mix it up. Many varieties of diffusers are available; follow diffuser manufacturer instructions for adding essential oils.

Candle diffuser. I did an informal poll of more than two thousand people, including my students and readers of my books, and the candle diffuser seems to be the most popular kind of diffuser. An inexpensive form of heat diffuser, a candle diffuser typically uses a tea-light candle to heat a small bowl made of a substance that is safe to use with essential oils, such as ceramic, glass, or soapstone. The small candle heats the bowl and voilà— scent is released into the air.

Evaporative diffuser. As the name indicates, this type of diffuser employs the use of evaporation. A fan in the diffuser blows air through a pad or filter that has a few drops of essential oil on it. The air blowing through the pad causes the essential oil to evaporate.

Heat diffuser. Like an evaporative diffuser, a heat diffuser uses evaporation as the dispersal method; however, heat is faster than evaporation when it comes to diffusing essential oils. A heat diffuser may use a candle or light bulb to warm an essential oil and release its scent.

Ultrasonic diffuser. Typically requiring the addition of water, an ultrasonic diffuser generates a fine mist and sends tiny oil particles into the air. A few drops of oil are added to the water in the device, making the diffuser economical to run. Some even have timers. Because it adds moisture to the air, this method of diffusion can be particularly beneficial during the dry winter months or in dry climates.

Nebulizing diffuser. Unlike an ultrasonic diffuser, a nebulizing diffuser doesn't need the addition of water but instead diffuses pure essential oil directly into the air by breaking it up into super-tiny molecules. This type of diffuser is considered superior because it releases the entire oil into the air in very fine particles. In fact, a nebulizing diffuser is thought to be the most effective and therapeutic kind of diffuser available.

Benefits of Using Essential Oils in a Diffuser

Diffusing essential oils does the following:

- Cleans and purifies the air, discouraging the growth of bacteria, mold, viruses, and other pathogens.
- Boosts the immune system and overall wellness.
- Helps to increase concentration and focus.
- Promotes feelings of peace and well-being by increasing the negative ions in the atmosphere.
- Positively affects mood and emotional health.
- Reduces anxiety and stress.
- Bonus! Makes your house smell wonderful.

Some Common Essential Oils

Essential oils come from various sources; accordingly, they feature an array of different scents and offer a range of therapeutic effects. Here are some common essential oils that are used in aromatherapy:

Basil (*Ocimum basilicum*). Basil essential oil is known to provide relief for nervous system disorders and mental exhaustion. (In fact, when I have been working too hard, I use basil essential oil combined with mandarin essential oil in a diffuser.) This oil is antibacterial and antiseptic; it calms the nerves, reduces spasms, and can also work as a stimulant and expectorant.

Bergamot (*Citrus bergamia*). Fresh and citrusy, bergamot lifts a dark mood and eases feelings of depression. It blends well with many oils, especially chamomile and all citrus oils.

Black pepper (*Piper nigrum*). Used in topical applications, black pepper essential oil is included in blends designed to relieve sore muscles, painful varicose veins, and muscular tension. It's good for promoting regional circulation.

Cedarwood (*Cedrus atlantica*). Relaxing and sedating, cedarwood essential oil helps to relieve anxiety. Considered an aphrodisiac by some, cedarwood enhances sensuality. It's often used in regenerative skin therapies in combination with jasmine or sandalwood. This woodsy oil blends well with citrus and floral oils.

Chamomile, Roman (*Anthemis nobilis*). Long used for skin and wound care, chamomile essential oil is beneficial in treating bruises, insect bites, psoriasis, sprains, and swelling. Because it's relaxing and reduces spasms, it's also helpful in treating muscle and nerve pain. For example, applying a chamomile compress to areas of nerve pain can offer relief.

Clary sage (*Salvia sclarea*). Found in many aromatherapy blends and in calming room sprays, clary sage essential oil is a favorite among aromatherapy enthusiasts. Sedating and relaxing, clary sage oil can cause mild euphoria, so it should be used carefully. It's more likely to cause motor impairment than any other essential oil, so some aromatherapists warn against using it with alcohol or drugs that cause similar effects.

Cypress (*Cupressus sempervirens*). Noted for its ability to heal wounds, soothe sore muscles, and reduce cramping, cypress essential oil has a number of beneficial properties. It's antibacterial, anti-inflammatory, and antiseptic; it works well as a deodorant, expectorant, sedative, and tonic.

Eucalyptus (*Eucalyptus globulus; Eucalyptus radiata*). Long used as a therapy for respiratory ailments, eucalyptus is a great essential oil for treating colds, congestion, flu, and sinus problems, including infections. It's antibacterial, antifungal, and antiseptic; it also relieves pain and spasms. In addition, it's a good treatment for wounds, although it may cause skin irritation.

Frankincense (*Boswellia carteri*). Soothing and relaxing, frankincense essential oil is popular for relieving anxiety and stress. As an expectorant, it's valuable in treating asthma and bronchitis. Used topically in a compress, lotion, or massage oil, it's an effective chest rub and antiseptic; it's also good for treating rheumatism and scars.

Geranium (*Pelargonium graveolens*). Geranium essential oil is frequently included in blends designed to alleviate depression or lift a dark mood. In addition, many people love the regenerative properties this oil offers in skin-care formulas. Recent research also has shown this oil's potential in treating and managing pain. For example, blended with a carrier oil or mixed into a salve, geranium essential oil can be helpful in treating nerve pain, neuropathy, and shingles.

Grapefruit (*Citrus paradisi*). Light and refreshing, grapefruit essential oil is one of my favorites. It's great for treating anxiety, irritability, and stress, especially for someone who is breaking an addiction or going through withdrawal. In addition, this oil is useful during times of hormonal upheaval and exhaustion—or when a lift in spirits is needed. It's antibacterial, antiseptic, astringent, restorative, and stimulating; it also aids depression and digestion.

Jasmine (*Jasminum grandiflorum*). Deeply relaxing, jasmine essential oil is also an aphrodisiac used to relieve sexual tension. In addition, it's wonderful for the skin, especially stressed or mature skin. It can be used to relieve pain, reduce inflammation, and promote menstrual flow.

Juniper (*Juniperus communis*). Known for giving gin its distinctive flavor, juniper also has many other uses. This essential oil is an astringent that is helpful for treating acne. In addition, it relieves pain and spasms, so it's used to treat sore joints and muscles. It's also an antimicrobial and sedative.

Lavender (*Lavandula angustifolia*). Lavender essential oil is beloved for its skin-healing properties in addition to its many other uses. In a diffuser blend, it can promote a calm, relaxing environment and lessen stress; it even relaxes and soothes infants. It's also earned a place in any first-aid kit because it can treat cuts and scrapes, insect bites, sore muscles, and sunburn. In addition, it's helpful in treating stress and tension. For example, a lavender compress can be used to relieve headaches, muscle pain, stress, and sunburn.

Lavender is considered one of the safest essential oils on the market. Some sources say it's okay to use lavender essential oil neat, or without dilution; however, to prevent reactions, I recommend that lavender essential oil always be diluted. Sensitivity can occur suddenly or after long-term use, and mixing lavender with a carrier oil can help prevent this.

Lemon (*Citrus limon*). A staple in many homes, lemon essential oil is used in a variety of household applications. It's an effective antifungal.

Mandarin (*Citrus reticulata*). Good at promoting sleep and relaxation and relieving insomnia and stress, mandarin essential oil is also an excellent essential oil for when you're feeling tired and sluggish. In addition, it's beneficial for skin issues, such as acne, aging skin, dull skin, oily skin, and scars.

Marjoram (*Origanum majorana*). Known for its sweet and camphoraceous scent, marjoram essential oil relieves pain and spasms and is soothing for strains as well as aching or cramping muscles. An effective expectorant, it can also be used to relieve coughs and colic. This oil also has analgesic, antiseptic, antiviral, bactericidal, fungicidal, and sedative actions.

Neroli (*Citrus aurantium*). Traditionally used to treat depression, stress, and other types of emotional upheaval, neroli essential oil is also beneficial for skin issues, including mature skin and stretch marks, and is often found in skin creams and oils. Obtained from orange blossoms, this essential oil is coveted for its ability to mix well with almost all other essential oils.

Oregano (*Origanum vulgare*). An effective antifungal and antimicrobial, oregano essential oil is valued for its effectiveness in treating skin ailments, including eczema and psoriasis.

Patchouli (*Pogostemon cablin*). Sometimes called the "hippie oil" and often remembered as the scent of the 1960s, Patchouli essential oil is an excellent base for an oil blend. Over time, its scent improves, its color changes, and it becomes richer.

Peppermint (*Mentha x piperita*). Peppermint essential oil has myriad uses. It's beneficial for fatigue, exhaustion, skin eruptions, sore muscles, and nausea. For example, a few drops of this essential oil on a handkerchief can be sniffed to help relieve nausea. Peppermint essential oil is also cooling and offers pain relief for chicken pox, insect bites, scabies, and shingles; it can even be applied to relieve toothaches. It can also promote urinary flow if a few drops are added to the toilet bowl. And finally, a few drops of peppermint and lavender essential oils can be added to laundry to eliminate unwanted odors.

Pine (*Pinus sylvestris*). We all know the scent of pine. Refreshing and invigorating, it's in the air and in our cleaning products. In fact, the smell of pine is associated with a fresh and clean house. Used in inhalation therapy, pine essential oil helps clear the sinuses. When included in a massage oil, it's effective in treating acute joint pain.

Rose petal (*Rosa damascena*). The delicate scent of rose is one of the most familiar in the world, and it's been valued for its sedative and aphrodisiac effects since the beginning of time. Rose essential oil is often found in facial oils and creams because it's both antibacterial and antiseptic.

Rosemary (*Rosmarinus officinalis*). A versatile essential oil to include in a first-aid kit, rosemary is antimicrobial, making it an excellent treatment for cuts and scrapes, and clears congestion. It's also useful for treating headaches in general and migraines in particular. A good way to treat a headache is to combine a few drops of rosemary essential oil with a carrier oil, such as vegetable oil, and massage this mixture into the temples. In addition, research has shown that the scent of rosemary essential oil can improve cognitive performance as well as mood.

Rosewood (*Aniba rosaeodora*). Known for its uplifting effect, rosewood essential oil is stimulating, relieves depression, and acts as an aphrodisiac. It's also a good oil to use on mature skin. Rosewood essential oil is antiseptic, bactericidal, deodorizing, and insecticidal.

Sandalwood (*Santalum album*). One of my favorite oils, sandalwood is, in a word, exotic. I often suggest sandalwood and rose essential oils for clients who want to relax and "get in the mood." When purchasing sandalwood essential oil, make sure it comes from a sustainable source.

Sweet orange (*Citrus sinensis*). Sweet orange essential oil is a light oil that is used in many everyday items, including air fresheners, cleaning products, and laundry soaps. Therapeutically, it alleviates feelings of anxiety and stress. For example, it's a good choice for children who are feeling insecure before a test. It's also effective for treating sadness and depression, including postpartum depression.

Tangerine (*Citrus reticulata*). I love the smell of citrus essential oils and especially tangerine. It has an uplifting effect for people who are feeling sluggish or worn down. This oil is antiseptic, relieves spasms, and is a sedative; for example, it's beneficial for stress and insomnia.

Tea tree (*Melaleuca alternifolia*). Tea tree is an extremely popular essential oil, with good reason; it's effective in addressing a wide range of issues. It can be used to treat candida, chicken pox, colds, cold sores, cuts and scrapes, flu, headaches, insect bites, and itchiness. Tea tree is well researched. For instance, one study found that a 5 percent tea tree oil gel made a significant difference in treating acne. Another study demonstrated that tea tree essential oil is great for treating athlete's foot. Because this oil can cause sensitivity when applied straight, I recommend always using it in a dilution. Tea tree essential oil is analgesic, antibacterial, antifungal, anti-inflammatory, antimicrobial, antiseptic, antiviral, fungicidal, and insecticidal; it also works as a decongestant, deodorant, and expectorant.

Vetiver (*Vetiveria zizanoides*). With its mellow and slightly earthy scent, vetiver essential oil is known for its anti-inflammatory, antiseptic, aphrodisiac, and sedative actions. This oil has a grounding and calming effect for many people. In addition, it's beneficial for dry skin, aching joints, and sore muscles.

Ylang-ylang (*Cananga odorata*). Ylang-ylang essential oil is considered relaxing, and it's useful for hormonal mood swings associated with premenstrual syndrome and menopause. In a diffuser blend, this essential oil can assist with feelings of angst, anxiety, and irritability. Also effective against depression, it's found in many antidepressant blends.

Essential Oil Safety

Essential oils, like any other substance that is used therapeutically, should be handled properly. Purchase them with care, use them with knowledge, and store them so they will last. Useful guidelines for buying, using, and storing essential oils follow.

Buying Essential Oils

Choosing an essential oil—or an essential oil company to purchase from— deserves careful consideration. My advice is to evaluate each essential oil individually; don't assume that if you like a certain essential oil company, you'll always prefer its oils. Although some people swear by one supplier, my essential oil cupboard is stocked with a variety of brands because I always take the time to research each individual essential oil I purchase. Fortunately, there is no shortage of reliable essential oil suppliers, and most will answer questions and welcome customer feedback.

Essential oils can be found in stores or online. The advantage of purchasing in a store, of course, is that you can smell and feel the essential oil before purchasing it. But there are other important considerations to keep in mind. Here are some tips on how to buy essential oils:

Do your homework. Before you buy it—and before you use it—read about the essential oil that interests you. Check a few sources to confirm it's the right choice to meet your needs.

Read the label. Make sure that what you're buying is an actual pure essential oil. The label should list only the common and botanical (or Latin) name of the essential oil; for example, sweet orange essential oil (*Citrus sinensis*) or bitter orange essential oil (*Citrus aurantium*). Sometimes an essential oil is bottled with a carrier oil; if so, the label should be marked accordingly. Keep this in mind when you intend to buy a blend or a diluted essential oil.

Be wary of labels that feature potentially confusing or misleading terms, such as "fragrance oil," "nature identical oil," "perfume oil," or "therapeutic oil." When such terms appear on labels, they signal that the bottle contents are not pure, single essential oils. In addition, be leery of terms such as "aromatherapy grade," "medical grade," and "therapeutic grade." There are no formal standards or "grades" used in the industry, so the inclusion of such terms on a label may be intentionally misleading.

Follow your nose. If you're purchasing an essential oil at a store, smell the oil sample and make sure you like it. If the scent turns you off, listen to your senses and find an alternative. The good news is that in almost all cases you can find a different essential oil to meet your needs. You can always revisit the essential oil you didn't like at a later date.

Your ability to identify a high-quality oil will develop over time, as you gain experience. Look for (or sniff for) an essential oil that smells like the plant it's distilled from. If you can detect anything else, such as chemicals or fillers, pass on purchasing that particular essential oil.

Feel the essential oil. When you're at a store looking at a sample, put a drop of essential oil on your finger and rub the oil between your finger and thumb. It should feel clean and not too oily. Some of the thicker, darker oils, such as patchouli and vetiver, can be more oily than lighter oils, such as lavender or sweet orange.

Pick proper packaging. Choose essential oils that are packaged in dark bottles. Amber is the darkest, and that's what I prefer, although you can also find cobalt blue, green, and violet bottles, which are acceptable. Make sure the bottles are topped with orifice reducers and caps—not droppers, which erode over time and allow air to enter the bottles. Always avoid essential oils sold in plastic or clear bottles.

Shop around. Essential oils aren't inexpensive. Look around online and in stores to get a feel for reasonable costs. If you see a price that seems too good to be true, it probably is. When purchasing online, make sure all the essential oils aren't priced the same. Uniform pricing is a red flag that the seller may not be reputable, because different varieties of essential oils simply should not cost the same (see box on opposite page).

Essential Oils Go to Market

In North America and all over the world, essential oils begin as a crop on a farm. The crop is harvested and transported to a distillation facility, where the essential oils are made. Some companies produce their product from seed to bottle, but many do not.

This final product is then sold in bulk quantities on the commodities market. Naturally, based on their ingredients and production factors, essential oils will vary in price and quality. Although some companies claim to offer "therapeutic grade" essential oils, this is just a marketing term. No official international distinctions, standards, or grades exist; no North American distinctions exist, for that matter.

There simply is no legal or industry standard definition of what a therapeutic grade essential oil is. Unfortunately, in the world of essential oils, no guaranteed standard exists, so it's important to shop discriminately.

Using Essential Oils Safely

When it comes to essential oil safety, I always advise erring on the side of caution. While this book is a guide to using aromatherapy at home, keep in mind that you can always consult a professional aromatherapist for help when necessary.

Avoid internal use. Don't use essential oils internally; that is, don't ingest them. Although some companies that sell essential oils advocate their internal use, this practice has not been proved to be safe. I never recommend internal use.

Always mix with a carrier oil. I've been using essential oils for over twenty-five years, and I never apply essential oils neat, or without dilution. I always use a carrier oil because I'm never sure how an essential oil will act or react with any person, even me, and using a carrier oil reduces the risk of a negative reaction. A carrier oil can be any nut, seed, or vegetable oil (see page 27).

Be aware of the potential for allergies and sensitivities. Essential oils can cause an allergic reaction or sensitivity. There are several steps you can take to prevent a reaction: never use undiluted essential oils (as described above), do a patch test (see box below), and alternate the essential oils you use so that a sensitivity doesn't develop.

If an allergic reaction occurs when an essential oil is used topically, remove as much of it as you can by wiping the skin with a cloth soaked in milk or vegetable oil. The essential oil will bond with the fat in the milk or oil. Follow that with a thorough washing or shower.

Patch Test

When I work with aromatherapy clients, I always suggest doing a patch test before using any essential oil. The simple instructions for doing a patch test on yourself follow:

• Apply 1 to 2 drops of the diluted essential oil inside the crease of your elbow.

• Cover the area with a bandage and keep it dry for 24 hours. Do not wash the area.

• If irritation, itching, redness, or swelling occurs, this essential oil may not be the one for you.

• Remember that if the essential oil doesn't cause a reaction for you, it may for someone else.

Pay attention to irritation. If irritation occurs, stop using the essential oil. Irritation can include feeling irritable or can refer to what's happening on the skin, such as contact dermatitis, hives, a rash, or redness. Irritation can occur with any application; if a diffused essential oil puts you in a bad mood, that's a negative reaction and reason to stop using that essential oil.

Less is more. Although people tend to think that more of a good thing can only be better, this is not the case when working with essential oils.

In fact, the opposite is true; it's always best to use the smallest effective amount. For example, if the recommended dosage is 5 drops, see if you get the same results with just 2 drops. Don't make a formula any stronger than necessary.

Keep away from flames. Remember that essential oils are flammable. Use caution when using them near an open flame, such as a candle diffuser.

Avoid mucus membranes. Don't use essential oils on or around the mucous membranes of the eyes, genitals, mouth, and nasal passages.

Consider special needs. Use appropriate caution when using essential oils with infants, children, pregnant women, and older adults. These groups may be much more sensitive to the effects of essential oils than a typical adult.

Essential Oil Storage and Equipment

Since essential oils can be expensive, it's important to store them with care. Here are some simple storage guidelines:

Proper containers. Make sure all essential oils are sold and stored in dark bottles with a tightly sealed cap. Droppers should never be left on the bottles to function as caps during storage.

Proper storage. Store all essential oils in a cool, dark place. Exposure to direct sunlight in particular or any light in general will speed up oxidation and break down the essential oil.

Shelf life. Most essential oils have a shelf life of two years. Some, such as citrus oils, keep for only one year. Pine and tea tree oil keep for about eighteen months. Patchouli and sandalwood keep a good bit longer than most, up to four years.

Mixing. Always mix essential oils with carrier oils (see page 27) in glass bottles or jars or porcelain or aluminum bottles (aluminum bottles must have a phenolic lining). Never use plastic, because essential oils can degrade it.

After putting the carrier oil in the bottle, use a dropper to add the essential oil or oils. I recommend that you use a separate dropper for every essential oil. Make sure you draw the essential oil only into the glass stem and not into the dropper's bulb. The bulb is rubber, and it will degrade and break down if exposed to essential oils over a prolonged period.

Cleaning. Use vodka or another alcohol to clean the droppers. Draw the vodka into the dropper and allow it to soak in the dropper. Alternatively, take the bulb off of the stem and let both pieces soak in white vinegar before rinsing with boiling water to sterilize.

Essential Oils to Avoid

The following essential oils are known to be unsafe, and trained aromatherapists avoid them. In most cases, you can find a safe alternative to any of the oils listed:

Ajowan (*Trachyspermum copticum*)

Almond, bitter (*Prunus dulcis* var. *amara*)

Arnica (*Arnica montana*)

Birch, sweet (*Betula lenta*)

Boldo leaf (*Peumus boldus*)

Broom, Spanish (*Spartium junceum*)

Calamus (*Acorus calamus* var. *angustatus*)

Camphor, brown (*Cinnamomum camphora*)

Camphor, yellow (*Cinnamomum camphora*)

Deer tongue (*Carphephorus odoratissimus*)

Garlic (*Allium sativum*)

Horseradish (*Armoracia rusticana*)

Jaborandi (*Pilocarpus jaborandi*)

Melilotus (*Melilotus officinalis*)

Mugwort (*Artemisia vulgaris*)

Mustard (*Brassica nigra*)

Onion (*Allium cepa*)

Pennyroyal (*Mentha pulegium*)

Rue (*Ruta graveolens*)

Sassafras (*Sassafras albidum*)

Tansy (*Tanacetum vulgare*)

Thuja (*Thuja occidentalis*)

Wintergreen (*Gaultheria procumbens*)

Wormseed (*Chenopodium ambrosioides* var. *anthelminticum*)

Wormwood (*Artemisia absinthium*)

Essential Oils to Avoid During Pregnancy

The following oils should be avoided during pregnancy:

Anise (*Pimpinella anisum*)

Basil (*Ocimum basilicum*)

Bay (*Pimenta racemosa*)

Bay laurel (*Laurus nobilis*)

Cedarwood, Atlas (*Cedrus atlantica*)

Cedarwood, Virginian (*Juniperus virginiana*)

Clary sage (*Salvia sclarea*)

Clove (*Eugenia caryophyllata*)

Cypress (*Cupressus sempervirens*)

Davana (*Artemisia pallens*)

Elemi (*Canarium luzonicum*)

Fennel (*Foeniculum vulgare*)

Geranium (*Pelargonium graveolens*)

Holy basil (*Ocimum gratissimum, Ocimum sanctum, Ocimum tenuiflorum*)

Hyssop (*Hyssopus officinalis*)

Jasmine (*Jasminum grandiflorum*)

Juniper (*Juniperus communis*)

Kanuka (*Leptospermum ericoides*)

Lavendin (*Lavandula hybrida*)

Linden blossom (*Tilia vulgaris*)

Marjoram (*Origanum majorana*)

May chang (*Litsea cubeba*)

Myrrh (*Commiphora myrrha*)

Nutmeg (*Myristica fragrans*)

Oakmoss (*Evernia prunastri*)

Oregano (*Origanum vulgare*)

Parsley (*Petroselinum sativum*)

Palo santo (*Bursera graveolens*)

Peppermint (*Mentha piperita*)

Peru balsam (*Myroxylon pereirae*)

Ravensara (*Ravensara aromatica*)

Rose, geranium (*Pelargonium roseum*)

Rosemary (*Rosmarinus officinalis*)

Sage (*Salvia officinalis*)

Sage, Dalmatian (*Salvia officinalis*)

Saro or **mandravasarotra** (*Cinnamosma fragrans*)

Spanish sage (*Salvia lavandulaefolia*)

Star anise (*Illicium verum*)

Tansy (*Tanacetum vulgare*)

Tansy, blue (*Tanacetum annuum*)

Thyme (*Thymus vulgaris*)

Yarrow (*Achillea millefolium*)

Blending Essential Oils: The Basics

If one essential oil is good, combining two or more can be better. Blend essential oils for their fragrance or therapeutic value, or both. Always follow safety tips (see page 19) when blending oils and creating aromatherapy applications.

Top, Middle, and Base Notes

The scent of a blend of essential oils changes over time. This is because different essential oils have varying evaporation rates. As the essential oils in the blend evaporate, the odor changes to reflect the aromas of the remaining oil or oils:

• Top notes evaporate in one to two hours. Top notes tend to be the primary or most noticeable scent you detect in a blend.

• Middle notes are slightly heavier and evaporate in two to four hours. These are often herbaceous scents.

• Base notes take longer to evaporate—sometimes several days.

Balancing a Blend

The trick to balancing a blend of essential oils is to know which families get along. That is, essential oils can be characterized into broad groups, or families, based on their aroma types. Essential oils in the same family typically blend well together. The following list shows which families blend well with each other:

• Exotic and spicy scents blend well with citrusy and floral scents.

• Flowery scents blend well with citrusy, spicy, and woodsy scents.

• Mint scents blend well with citrusy, earthy, herbaceous, and woodsy scents.

• Woodsy and outdoorsy scents generally blend well with all other families.

It's easy to experiment with blending. Take a few drops of three different essential oils and smell them individually, then mix them together. How does the combination differ from the original essential oils? How does the scent change over time as the essential oils begin to evaporate? Several hours can make quite a difference in the scent of any essential oil blend. (See "Top, Middle, and Base Notes," above.)

The following is a common grouping of essential oil families:

Citrusy. Citrusy oils are often top notes, evaporate pretty quickly, and blend well with most scents. The most popular citrus essential oils are grapefruit, lemon, lemon balm, lemongrass, lime, mandarin, orange, and tangerine.

Earthy. Earthy scents, which are typically base notes, bring to mind fresh air, earth, and water. These include oakmoss, patchouli, and vetiver.

Exotic. Typically middle and base notes, exotic essential oils are all lovely and include ginger (*Zingiber officinale*), patchouli, sandalwood, and ylang-ylang.

Flowery. Floral scents are often top notes or middle notes. These include jasmine, lavender, neroli, palmarosa (*Cymbopogon martini*), rose, and ylang-ylang.

Herbaceous. Made from herbs, these essential oils have a distinctively "green" scent and include basil, clary sage, hyssop, and marjoram.

Medicinal or camphorous. Usually top and middle notes, these essential oils include eucalyptus, ravensara, rosemary, and tea tree.

Mint family (*Lamiaceae family*). Mint is one of the most familiar essential oils and includes lavender, peppermint, and spearmint (*Mentha spicata*). These tend to be top and middle notes.

Spicy. Warm, often exotic, and reminiscent of certain kitchen spices, these scents include allspice (*Pimenta officinalis*), cardamom (*Elettaria cardamomum*), cassia (*Cinnamomum cassia*), clove, and nutmeg.

Woodsy. Woodsy essential oils are middle or base notes and always bring nature and outdoors to mind. These include cedarwood, cypress, pine, and spruce (*Picea mariana*).

Easy Ways to Use Essential Oils

One of the simplest and most effective ways to receive the benefits of essential oils is to smell them. Open the cap and take a sniff. Or put a few drops on a handkerchief that you can carry with you. You can use essential oils this way anytime, anywhere. Here are two other easy applications that will allow you to enjoy essential oils with almost no effort:

- Make a natural air freshener spray to use at home, at work, or in the car. Put 2 ounces of pure water in a mist spray bottle and add 50 to 75 drops of an essential oil. Shake well before spraying into the air. I use this application in the car and in the living room, places that tend to get a little stinky thanks to my two sons.
- Add 25 drops of one or more essential oils to a bowl of potpourri that has lost its scent. Or create your own potpourri by adding drops of an essential oil to dried leaves, flowers, and so on. Mix together in a container, cover tightly, and store for several days to allow the potpourri to absorb the essential oil.

Essentials for Making Blends

In addition to the essential oils themselves, only a few pieces of equipment and ingredients are needed to make aromatherapy blends. Most are items that you may already have at home, and all are inexpensive.

Carrier oils. Used in liniments, massage oils, and other topical applications, carrier oils are used to "carry" the essential oil. Carrier oils can be any nut, seed, or vegetable oils. Apricot kernel oil, olive oil, and sweet almond oil are some examples. Carrier oils are added only after the essential oils are mixed and when you're ready to use the blend.

Liquids. Used in liniments, sprays, and toners, various liquids can be added to essential oils. These include water, witch hazel, or a food-grade alcohol, such as vodka.

Dropper bottles or glass jars. Essential oils are volatile and begin to evaporate upon contact with the air, so it's advisable to immediately put the cap on the bottle or jar after putting in the essential oils. Add a few drops at a time to the bottle or jar, put on the cap, and gently swish the essential oils to mix.

Droppers or pipettes. Droppers are slender glass tubes that have a rubber bulb at one end. They're used for transferring liquids or essential oils to a bottle or jar. Pipettes are thin glass tubes that may incorporate a glass bulb at one end; they also can be used for this purpose. At about ten cents apiece, pipettes are affordable and can be reused when cleaned properly. Droppers are more expensive but are also reusable when cleaned properly.

How to Make an Essential Oil Blend

When blending essential oils for use in aromatherapy, first determine the types of essential oils that may be useful by researching various therapeutic actions and their effects. List the required actions desired, such as reduce pain, and the supportive actions desired, such as enhance mood. Then select the essential oils that meet your needs. Use your research to determine the number of drops of each essential oil to start with.

Use a dropper or pipette to put the drops of essential oil in the dropper bottle or jar. Start with equal amounts of the essential oils and increase them one at a time if desired. Put on the cap and gently swish the bottle in a circular motion to mix. Remove the cap to test the fragrance and effect. If desired, use scent strips (neutral blotter strips that are used for testing a fragrance) to test the blend. Put a few drops on a strip and smell away. When you're ready to use the essential oil blend, add the carrier oil (see page 27).

Basic Methods for Making Aromatherapy Applications

Before trying the recipe (pages 31 to 46) for any aromatherapy application, review the following section to become familiar with the primary methods.

The recipes will provide specifics, such as the types and amounts of the ingredients. To mix the application, refer back to this section.

Body Sprays

To make a body spray, put the essential oils in a glass spray bottle (a typical amount is 30 to 40 drops of essential oils in a 4-ounce glass spray bottle, but recipes may vary). Add enough base liquid, such as water or vodka, to fill the bottle. Vodka or another alcohol will act as a preservative. Put the spray cap on the bottle and shake well to combine.

Room Sprays

Similar to body sprays, room sprays tend to be more concentrated. To make a room spray, combine essential oils with a food-grade alcohol, such as vodka, in a glass or metal spray bottle that can be set to distribute a fine mist. Shake well to combine.

Bath Oils

An easy way to enjoy aromatherapy is to add essential oils to a bath. All you need per bath is 1 teaspoon (5 ml) to 1 tablespoon (15 ml) of an essential oil or blend. A little oil goes a really long way. Make sure the essential oil or blend is adequately dispersed in the water.

Blended and Massage Oils

Blended and massage oils are made with a carrier oil (see page 27) and essential oils. Put all the ingredients in a glass bottle and shake well to combine. If the massage oil blend is too strong, add more carrier oil to dilute. If the massage oil isn't potent enough, add a few more drops of one of the essential oils. Store in a tightly sealed glass bottle.

Diffuser Blends

Many of the recipes for blended and massage oils in this book can be used as diffuser blends if the carrier oil is omitted. It's essential to check the diffuser manufacturer's instructions when using essential oil blends in a diffuser; one important consideration is the amount of oil that can be safely used in the diffuser at one time. The recommended blends in this book (see pages 31 to 46) may produce amounts that are too great to be diffused at once. Here are a few popular essential oils to use in diffuser blends:

- Cedarwood, chamomile, clary sage, geranium, juniper, lavender, marjoram, and tangerine can help to relieve stress.
- Cedarwood, chamomile, clary sage, cypress, frankincense, geranium, juniper, lavender, rosewood, sandalwood, tangerine, and ylang-ylang can help reduce tension.

Creams and Lotions

Start with a favorite cream or lotion, preferably unscented. Thoroughly mix in the essential oil or blend (a typical amount is 15 to 30 drops of essential oils to each ounce of cream or lotion, but recipes may vary). Test before using. The fatty base of some creams or lotions may make an essential oil feel stronger; if so, try adding a bit more cream or lotion to dilute. Store in a tightly sealed glass bottle or jar.

Liniments

Liniments are made with food-grade alcohol, such as vodka, or witch hazel and essential oils. Do not use rubbing alcohol to make a liniment. Put all the ingredients in a glass bottle and shake well to combine. Store in a tightly sealed glass bottle.

Simple Salves

Salves are made with both a carrier oil and a hard wax or oil, such as beeswax, a vegetarian wax, or coconut oil. The ratio of ingredients in a recipe can vary, but here is a general formula: to make 2 cups (500 ml) of salve, combine 2 cups (500 ml) of a carrier oil with 1.5 ounces or 3 tablespoons (45 ml) of wax.

Put the carrier oil and wax in a small saucepan and warm over low heat, stirring until all the wax is melted. Stir in the essential oils (and any herbs, if using). Pour into a glass bottle or container. When the salve cools, if it seems too hard, repeat the process and add more oil. Similarly, if it seems too soft, add more wax. Store in a tightly sealed glass bottle or container. Following are examples of essential oils that work well in salves:

- Bergamot, chamomile (German and Roman), frankincense, geranium, and neroli essential oils can help to relieve stress.
- Black pepper, clary sage, peppermint, and chamomile essential oils are good for muscle aches and pains.
- Geranium, lavender, palmarosa, rose, and rosewood essential oils have healing effects.

Aromatherapy Applications for Physical Well-Being

ANTIFUNGALS

Antifungal Oil

1 ounce carrier oil (see page 27)
10 drops tea tree essential oil
5 drops chamomile essential oil
5 drops lavender essential oil

Follow the method for making blended oils, page 29. Apply to the affected area 2 or 3 times a day.

Oregano Antifungal Powder

1 cup (250 ml) cornstarch
10 drops oregano essential oil
10 drops tea tree essential oil

Put the cornstarch in a small jar and add the essential oils. Put the lid on the jar and shake to mix well. Let sit for 1 week before using.

ARTHRITIS AND SORE MUSCLES

Acute Joint Pain Massage Oil

2 ounces carrier oil
    (see page 27)
10 drops juniper essential oil
2 drops rosemary essential oil
1 drop pine essential oil

Follow the method for making massage oils, page 29. Massage into the affected areas.

Arthritis Massage Oil

4 ounces sweet almond oil,
    apricot kernel oil, or other
    carrier oil (see page 27)
10 drops black pepper essential oil
10 drops fennel essential oil
10 drops juniper essential oil
10 drops peppermint essential oil

Follow the method for making massage oils, page 29. Massage into sore and arthritic joints.

Black Pepper Muscle Oil

½ cup (125 ml) carrier oil
  (see page 27)
40 drops black pepper essential
  oil
10 drops clary sage essential oil
10 drops lavender essential oil

Follow the method for making blended oils, page 29. Apply to sore muscles.

Note: This is a potent blend, so if it's too strong, add more carrier oil.

Muscle Pain Liniment

½ cup (125 ml) vodka
1 teaspoon (5 ml) peppermint,
  eucalyptus, or rosemary
  essential oil

Follow the method for making liniments, page 30.

Note: Try using less essential oil at first to see if a smaller amount is effective for you.

Variation: If desired, use a blend of essential oils, but keep in mind that the final ratio should be no more than 1 teaspoon (5 ml) of essential oils per 1 cup (250 ml) of vodka.

Peppermint Muscle and Joint Rub

1 tablespoon (15 ml) cream or
  lotion
10 drops peppermint essential oil

Follow the method for blending creams, page 30. Apply to the affected areas.

Note: This blend is strong and will really penetrate sore muscles.

Variation: Use 5 drops of peppermint essential oil and 5 drops of black pepper essential oil.

Tendonitis Massage Oil

2 tablespoons (30 ml) sweet
  almond oil, apricot kernel oil,
  or other carrier oil
  (see page 27)
12 drops peppermint essential oil
10 drops eucalyptus essential oil
10 drops rosemary essential oil

Follow the method for making massage oils, page 29. Massage into affected hands, wrists, and other joints. Apply this massage oil after treating the affected area with a cold compress.

BACKACHE

Backache Massage Oil

2 ounces carrier oil (see page 27)
10 drops peppermint essential oil
5 drops juniper essential oil
2 drops lavender essential oil

Follow the method for making massage oils, page 29. This is wonderful when used on the lower back. Massage firmly into the sacrum, lower back, and upper buttocks.

BASIC BODY CARE

Deodorant Spray

1 ounce vodka or witch hazel
40 drops bergamot essential oil
20 drops clary sage essential oil
20 drops lavender essential oil
20 drops tea tree essential oil

Follow the method for making body sprays, page 29. Combine all the ingredients in a 4-ounce glass spray bottle, then add enough water to fill the bottle. Put on the spray cap and shake well.

Hippie Body Deodorant Spray

1 ounce vodka or witch hazel
40 drops patchouli essential oil
20 drops mandarin essential oil
10 drops rose essential oil
10 drops sandalwood essential oil

Follow the method for making body sprays, page 29. Combine all the ingredients in a 4-ounce glass spray bottle, then add enough water to fill the bottle. Put on the spray cap and shake well.

COLD AND FLU

Cold and Flu Diffuser Blend

10 drops eucalyptus essential oil
10 drops orange essential oil
8 drops rosewood essential oil
7 drops pine essential oil
5 drops ginger essential oil
5 drops basil essential oil

Follow the method for making blended oils, page 29. Use per the diffuser manufacturer's instructions.

Variation: Use as an inhalation (see page 9) or add 2 to 4 drops to a bath.

Common Cold Massage Oil

1 teaspoon (5 ml) carrier oil
   (see page 27)
2 drops eucalyptus essential oil
2 drops lemon essential oil
2 drops rosemary essential oil

Follow the method for making massage oils, page 29. Massage into the chest, neck, and sinus area.

Expectorant Rub

½ cup (125 ml) coconut oil
10 drops basil essential oil
10 drops eucalyptus essential oil
10 drops tea tree essential oil

Follow the method for making blended oils, page 29. Rub into the chest to relieve chest congestion.

Tea Tree Cold and Flu Room Spray

2 tablespoons (30 ml) vodka
40 drops tea tree essential oil

Follow the method for making room sprays, page 29. Put the ingredients in a 4-ounce glass spray bottle, then add enough water to fill the bottle. Put on the spray cap and shake well.

Note: This blend is good for cleaning the air when cold and flu are present and can also be misted on bedding, doorknobs, toilet seats, and other surfaces.

HEADACHE

Headache Inhalation

Rock salt
3 drops lavender essential oil
3 drops peppermint essential oil
3 drops rosemary essential oil

Put a few large grains of rock salt in a 1- or 2-ounce bottle and add the essential oils. Put on the cap and shake to combine.

Gastric Headache Massage Oil

2 drops peppermint essential oil
1 drop lavender essential oil
1 drop rosemary essential oil

Combine the essential oils in a small glass bottle. Massage into the back of the neck.

Variation: Put 1 drop of the mixture on a tissue and inhale. Alternatively, use 3 to 5 drops in an over-the-bowl steam application (see page 9). The mixture may also be used as a diffuser blend.

Headache Massage Oil

3 drops lavender essential oil
1 drop peppermint essential oil
1 drop vegetable oil or other
   carrier oil (see page 27)

Combine the essential oils and carrier oil in a small glass bottle. Massage into the temples, the base of the skull, and along the hairline to relieve headache.

Variation: Omit the carrier oil and use as a diffuser blend.

MENSTRUAL CRAMPS AND PMS

Menstrual Cramp Massage Oil

¼ cup (60 ml) carrier oil
   (see page 27)
6 drops basil essential oil
4 drops lemongrass essential oil
4 drops marjoram essential oil

Follow the method for making massage oils, page 29. Massage into the lower abdomen as needed to relieve cramps.

Variation: Omit the carrier oil to use as a diffuser or inhalation blend.

PMS Diffuser Blend

3 drops sweet orange essential oil
2 drops clary sage essential oil
2 drops rosewood essential oil

Follow the method for making blended oils, page 29. Use per the diffuser manufacturer's instructions.

INSOMNIA

Insomnia Diffuser Blend

15 drops orange essential oil
10 drops chamomile essential oil
10 drops lavender essential oil
10 drops tangerine essential oil
8 drops clary sage essential oil
5 drops sandalwood essential oil
3 drops ylang-ylang essential oil

Follow the method for making blended oils, page 29. Use per the diffuser manufacturer's instructions.

Sweet Dreams Hand Cream

2 ounces thick, unscented
   hand cream
10 drops lavender essential oil
5 drops sweet orange essential oil

Follow the method for making creams, page 30. Rub into hands at bedtime.

Sweetest Dreams Massage Oil

¼ cup (60 ml) coconut oil or
   other carrier oil (see page 27)
5 drops neroli essential oil
4 drops clary sage essential oil
3 drops ylang-ylang essential oil
2 drops patchouli essential oil

Follow the method for making massage oils, page 29. Massage slowly and softly into the skin at bedtime.

ENERGY AND REVITALIZATION

Energizing Massage Oil

2 ounces carrier oil (see page 27)
10 drops grapefruit essential oil
10 drops sweet orange essential oil

Follow the method for making massage oils, page 29. Massage on the back of the neck and knees for an uplifted feeling.

Relaxing Body Powder

½ cup (125 ml) arrowroot starch
½ cup (125 ml) cornstarch
10 drops clary sage essential oil
10 drops lavender essential oil
10 drops sweet orange essential oil

Put the arrowroot starch and cornstarch in a small jar and add the essential oils. Put the lid on the jar. Shake to mix well. Let sit for 1 week before using.

RELAXATION

Deep Breathing Massage Oil

4 ounces carrier oil (see page 27)
10 drops clary sage essential oil
10 drops eucalyptus essential oil
10 drops lavender essential oil

Follow the method for making massage oils, page 29. Massage into the chest and upper back to promote deep breathing and relaxation.

Relaxation Diffuser Blend

7 drops mandarin essential oil
7 drops clary sage essential oil
5 drops lavender essential oil

Follow the method for making blended oils, page 29. Use per the diffuser manufacturer's instructions.

Relaxation Inhalation

Rock salt
3 drops clary sage essential oil
3 drops lavender essential oil
3 drops neroli essential oil

Put a few large grains of rock salt in a 1- or 2-ounce bottle and add the essential oils. Put on the cap and shake to combine.

Relaxation and Rest Body or Room Spray

15 drops clary sage essential oil
15 drops lavender essential oil
12 drops chamomile essential oil

Follow the method for making body sprays, page 29. Combine all the ingredients in a 4-ounce glass bottle, then add enough water to fill the bottle. Put on the spray cap and shake well.

Restlessness with Anxiety Diffuser Blend

10 drops myrrh essential oil
10 drops vetiver essential oil
5 drops sweet orange essential oil

Follow the method for making blended oils, page 29. Use per the diffuser manufacturer's instructions.

Revitalizing Bath Oil

½ cup (125 ml) carrier oil
20 drops geranium essential oil
10 drops clary sage essential oil
10 drops lemon essential oil

Follow the method for making blended oils, page 29. Add 1 to 2 teaspoons (5 to 10 ml) to the bath.

SKIN CARE

Mature-Skin Face Cream

3 tablespoons (45 ml) rose hip
  seed oil
2 drops frankincense essential oil
2 drops rose essential oil
1 vitamin E capsule

Follow the method for making
blended oils, page 29. Apply to face
and smooth over problem areas.
Use just a dab at a time.

Note: Rose hip seed oil is an excellent carrier oil to use on mature
skin, dry skin, or scar tissue.

Variation: Replace the frankincense essential oil with cedarwood,
lavender, or sandalwood essential
oils. Alternatively, replace both the
frankincense and rose essential oils
with cedarwood and grapefruit or
lavender essential oils, or clary sage
and patchouli essential oils.

Rose Face Cream

2 ounces unscented face cream
10 drops rose essential oil
2 drops vitamin E oil

Follow the method for making
creams, page 30. If you have sensitive skin, try using less rose essential oil, starting with 3 to 5 drops
and adding more as tolerated.

Variation: Use neroli essential oil
in place of rose essential oil, or use
half of each.

Neroli Body Cream

3 ounces unscented body cream
15 drops neroli essential oil
5 drops rose essential oil
5 drops sandalwood essential oil

Follow the method for making
creams, page 30. Use as needed.

Skin-Refreshing Body Spray

1.5 ounces vodka
1.5 ounces water
10 drops mandarin essential oil
10 drops patchouli essential oil
10 drops sweet orange essential oil
5 drops clary sage essential oil

Follow the method for making body
sprays, page 29. Combine all the ingredients in a 4-ounce glass spray
bottle.

Stretch Mark Massage Oil

1 cup (250 ml) cocoa butter,
  melted
3 tablespoons (45 ml) wheat
germ oil
2 tablespoons (30 ml) flaxseed oil
2 tablespoons (30 ml) rose hip
  seed oil
1 tablespoon (15 ml) borage oil
12 drops lavender essential oil
10 drops neroli essential oil
6 drops vetiver essential oil

Follow the method for making massage oils, page 29. Let cool to a comfortable temperature before using.
Massage into breasts and belly 1 or
2 times a day.

Aromatherapy Applications for Emotional and Mental Well-Being

ANXIETY

Anxiety Room Spray

20 drops ylang-ylang essential oil
10 drops clary sage essential oil
10 drops rose essential oil

Follow the method for making room sprays, page 29. Combine all the ingredients in a 2-ounce glass spray bottle. Spray as needed.

Anxiety Diffuser Blend 1

5 drops cedarwood essential oil
5 drops clary sage essential oil
5 drops tangerine essential oil

Anxiety Diffuser Blend 2

6 drops sandalwood essential oil
5 drops frankincense essential oil
5 drops lavender essential oil
3 drops marjoram essential oil

Follow the method for making blended oils, page 29. Use per the diffuser manufacturer's instructions.

BURNOUT AND EXHAUSTION

Energy-Boosting Room Spray

14 drops orange essential oil
10 drops grapefruit essential oil
10 drops lime essential oil
10 drops rosemary essential oil

Follow the method for making body sprays, page 29. Combine all the ingredients in a 4-ounce glass bottle, then add enough water to fill the bottle. Put on the spray cap and shake well.

Variation: Without adding any water, use in a diffuser per the manufacturer's instructions.

Calming Diffuser Blend

3 drops cedarwood essential oil
3 drops clary sage essential oil
2 drops mandarin essential oil

Follow the method for making blended oils, page 29. Use per the diffuser manufacturer's instructions.

Variation: To make a room spray, follow the method for making room sprays, page 29.

Burnout Diffuser Blend

15 drops frankincense essential oil
5 drops tangerine essential oil
4 drops sandalwood essential oil

Follow the method for making blended oils, page 29. Use per the diffuser manufacturer's instructions.

Exhaustion from Overwork Diffuser Blend

20 drops clary sage essential oil
10 drops orange essential oil

Follow the method for making blended oils, page 29. Use per the diffuser manufacturer's instructions.

Mental Fatigue Diffuser Blend

10 drops frankincense essential oil
10 drops lavender essential oil
5 drops rosemary essential oil
5 drops rosewood essential oil
5 drops spearmint essential oil

Follow the method for making blended oils, page 29. Use per the diffuser manufacturer's instructions.

Note: This blend is especially helpful for emotionally exhausted parents.

Uplifting Room Spray for New Mothers

20 drops orange essential oil
15 drops grapefruit essential oil
10 drops ylang-ylang essential oil
5 drops mandarin essential oil

Follow the method for making room sprays, page 29. Combine all the ingredients in a 4-ounce glass spray bottle, then add enough water to fill the bottle. Spray as needed.

Note: This blend is particularly good for women during the postpartum period, but it also can provide a lift to anyone, anytime.

FEAR AND WORRY

Fear-of-Failure Diffuser Blend

10 drops lavender essential oil
10 drops sandalwood essential oil
10 drops ylang-ylang essential oil

Follow the method for making blended oils, page 29. Use per the diffuser manufacturer's instructions.

Worry Diffuser Blend

15 drops chamomile essential oil
15 drops juniper essential oil
5 drops clary sage essential oil

Follow the method for making blended oils, page 29. Use per the diffuser manufacturer's instructions.

Worry about the Future Diffuser Blend

10 drops sandalwood essential oil
10 drops lavender essential oil
5 drops clary sage essential oil

Follow the method for making blended oils, page 29. Use per the diffuser manufacturer's instructions.

Worry about the Past Diffuser Blend

10 drops frankincense essential oil
5 drops mandarin essential oil

Follow the method for making blended oils, page 29. Use per the diffuser manufacturer's instructions.

GRIEF AND SADNESS

Grief Diffuser Blend

10 drops clary sage essential oil
10 drops marjoram essential oil
10 drops orange essential oil

Follow the method for making blended oils, page 29. Use per the diffuser manufacturer's instructions.

Grief over Long-Ago Events Diffuser Blend

15 drops grapefruit essential oil
10 drops tangerine essential oil
5 drops ravensara essential oil

Follow the method for making blended oils, page 29. Use per the diffuser manufacturer's instructions.

Hopelessness Diffuser Blend

10 drops mandarin essential oil
10 drops tangerine essential oil
5 drops orange essential oil

Follow the method for making blended oils, page 29. Use per the diffuser manufacturer's instructions.

Sadness Diffuser Blend 1

12 drops marjoram essential oil
10 drops orange essential oil
7 drops mandarin essential oil

Sadness Diffuser Blend 2

10 drops bergamot essential oil
5 drops cypress essential oil
5 drops pine essential oil
5 drops rosemary essential oil

Follow the method for making blended oils, page 29. Use per the diffuser manufacturer's instructions.

HYSTERIA

Hysteria Diffuser Blend 1

10 drops chamomile essential oil
10 drops lavender essential oil
5 drops peppermint essential oil

Hysteria Diffuser Blend 2

10 drops chamomile essential oil
10 drops marjoram essential oil
10 drops lemon balm essential oil
 (*Melissa officinalis*)

Follow the method for making blended oils, page XX. Use per the diffuser manufacturer's instructions.

NEGATIVE EMOTIONS

Impatience Diffuser Blend

10 drops chamomile essential oil
10 drops lavender essential oil
10 drops ylang-ylang essential oil

Follow the method for making blended oils, page 29. Use per the diffuser manufacturer's instructions.

Insecurity Diffuser Blend 1

10 drops bergamot essential oil
10 drops juniper essential oil
5 drops sandalwood essential oil

Insecurity Diffuser Blend 2

10 drops geranium essential oil
5 drops jasmine essential oil
5 drops patchouli essential oil
5 drops vetiver essential oil

Follow the method for making blended oils, page 29. Use per the diffuser manufacturer's instructions.

Irritability Diffuser Blend

15 drops chamomile essential oil
5 drops cypress essential oil
5 drops lavender essential oil
5 drops sandalwood essential oil

Follow the method for making blended oils, page 29. Use per the diffuser manufacturer's instructions.

Irritability Room Spray

1 ounce vodka
20 drops lemon essential oil
20 drops grapefruit essential oil
10 drops sweet orange essential oil

Follow the method for making room sprays, page 29.

Jealousy Diffuser Blend 1

10 drops cypress essential oil
10 drops ylang-ylang essential oil
5 drops lemon essential oil

Jealousy Diffuser Blend 2

10 drops cedarwood essential oil
10 drops helichrysum essential oil
(*Helichrysum italicum*)
10 drops palmarosa essential oil

Follow the method for making blended oils, page 29. Use per the diffuser manufacturer's instructions.

Resentment Diffuser Blend 1

10 drops clary sage essential oil
10 drops lemon essential oil

Resentment Diffuser Blend 2

10 drops sandalwood essential oil
5 drops helichrysum essential oil
5 drops rose essential oil
5 drops ylang-ylang essential oil

Follow the method for making blended oils, page 29. Use per the diffuser manufacturer's instructions.

TROUBLING THOUGHTS

Negative Thoughts Diffuser Blend

20 drops clary sage essential oil
15 drops lavender essential oil

Follow the method for making blended oils, page 29. Use per the diffuser manufacturer's instructions.

Racing Thoughts Diffuser Blend

22 drops clary sage essential oil
12 drops neroli essential oil

Follow the method for making blended oils, page 29. Use per the diffuser manufacturer's instructions.

Restless Thoughts Diffuser Blend

25 drops chamomile essential oil
10 drops clary sage essential oil

Follow the method for making blended oils, page 29. Use per the diffuser manufacturer's instructions.

Scattered Thoughts Diffuser Blend

15 drops cedarwood essential oil
5 drops grapefruit essential oil

Follow the method for making blended oils, page 29. Use per the diffuser manufacturer's instructions.

Unclear Thoughts Diffuser Blend 1

15 drops eucalyptus essential oil
15 drops grapefruit essential oil

Unclear Thoughts Diffuser Blend 2

10 drops lemon essential oil
10 drops peppermint essential oil
10 drops rosemary essential oil

Follow the method for making blended oils, page 29. Use per the diffuser manufacturer's instructions.

PANIC ATTACKS

Panic Attack Diffuser Blend 1

10 drops clary sage essential oil
5 drops frankincense essential oil
5 drops lavender essential oil

Panic Attack Diffuser Blend 2

5 drops chamomile essential oil
5 drops rose essential oil
5 drops vetiver essential oil
5 drops ylang-ylang essential oil

Follow the method for making blended oils, page 29. Use per the diffuser manufacturer's instructions.

NERVOUS EXHAUSTION

Nervous Exhaustion Diffuser Blend 1

10 drops chamomile essential oil
10 drops clary sage essential oil
5 drops juniper essential oil

Nervous Exhaustion Diffuser Blend 2

15 drops basil essential oil
10 drops pine essential oil

Nervous Exhaustion Diffuser Blend 3

10 drops clary sage essential oil
10 drops rosemary essential oil
5 drops pine essential oil

Nervous Exhaustion Diffuser Blend 4

15 drops lavender essential oil
10 drops peppermint essential oil

Nervous Exhaustion Diffuser Blend 5

10 drops clary sage essential oil
10 drops vetiver essential oil
5 drops chamomile essential oil

Follow the method for making blended oils, page 29. Use per the diffuser manufacturer's instructions.

Overactive Mind Diffuser Blend

10 drops chamomile essential oil
10 drops lavender essential oil
5 drops marjoram essential oil

Follow the method for making blended oils, page 29. Use per the diffuser manufacturer's instructions.

Overburdened Diffuser Blend

15 drops rosewood essential oil
10 drops sandalwood essential oil

Follow the method for making blended oils, page 29. Use per the diffuser manufacturer's instructions.

Lack of Concentration Diffuser Blend 1

15 drops rosemary essential oil
10 drops cedarwood essential oil
5 drops eucalyptus essential oil

Lack of Concentration Diffuser Blend 2

15 drops rosemary essential oil
8 drops lemon essential oil
8 drops ylang-ylang essential oil
4 drops basil essential oil

Follow the method for making blended oils, page 29. Use per the diffuser manufacturer's instructions.

OVERCOMING OBSTACLES

Coping with New Responsibilities Diffuser Blend

20 drops rosemary essential oil
10 drops cedarwood essential oil
10 drops cypress essential oil
5 drops orange essential oil

Follow the method for making blended oils, page 29. Use per the diffuser manufacturer's instructions.

Note: This application is great for new moms and dads.

Variation: Follow the method for making room sprays, page 29. Combine all the ingredients in a 4-ounce glass bottle, then add enough water to fill the bottle. Put on the spray cap and shake well.

Difficulty Adjusting to Change Diffuser Blend

10 drops clary sage essential oil
5 drops lavender essential oil
5 drops tangerine essential oil

Follow the method for making blended oils, page 29. Use per the diffuser manufacturer's instructions.

STRESS

Stress Diffuser Blend 1

20 drops tangerine essential oil
10 drops lavender essential oil

Stress Diffuser Blend 2

10 drops cedarwood essential oil
10 drops juniper essential oil
10 drops marjoram essential oil

Stress Diffuser Blend 3

10 drops chamomile essential oil
10 drops clary sage essential oil
10 drops geranium essential oil

Stress Diffuser Blend 4

20 drops lavender essential oil
5 drops marjoram essential oil
5 drops tangerine essential oil

Follow the method for making blended oils, page 29. Use per the diffuser manufacturer's instructions.

TENSION

Tension Diffuser Blend 1

12 drops cedarwood essential oil
10 drops sandalwood essential oil
10 drops tangerine essential oil

Tension Diffuser Blend 2

15 drops lavender essential oil
10 drops chamomile essential oil
10 drops clary sage essential oil

Tension Diffuser Blend 3

15 drops rosewood essential oil
10 drops frankincense essential oil
10 drops sandalwood essential oil

Follow the method for making blended oils, page 29. Use per the diffuser manufacturer's instructions.

Aromatherapy Applications for Setting or Changing the Mood

UPLIFTING MOOD

Mood-Lightening Salve

½ cup (125 ml) coconut oil, melted
10 drops geranium essential oil
5 drops bergamot essential oil
5 drops rose essential oil

Follow the method for making salves, page 30. Let cool completely before applying.

Mood-Lifting Inhalation

Rock salt
3 drops bergamot essential oil
3 drops black pepper essential oil
3 drops mandarin essential oil

Put a few large grains of rock salt in a 1- or 2-ounce bottle and add the essential oils. Put on the cap and shake to combine.

SENSUAL MOOD

Romance Inhalation

Rock salt
3 drops jasmine essential oil
3 drops sandalwood essential oil
2 drops rose or sweet orange essential oil

Put a few large grains of rock salt in a 1- or 2-ounce bottle and add the essential oils. Put on the cap and shake to combine.

Sensual Bath Oil

½ cup (125 ml) carrier oil (see page 27)
20 drops jasmine essential oil
10 drops rose essential oil
10 drops sweet orange essential oil

Follow the method for making blended oils, page 29. Add 1 to 2 teaspoons (5 to 10 ml) to the bath.

Note: Although this is a good bath oil to use when you want to feel sexy and get "in the mood," it also promotes relaxation.

Sexy Body Powder

½ cup (125 ml) arrowroot starch
½ cup (125 ml) cornstarch
10 drops jasmine essential oil
10 drops rose essential oil
10 drops sandalwood essential oil

Put the arrowroot starch and cornstarch in a small jar and add the essential oils. Put the lid on the jar and shake to mix well. Let sit for 1 week before using.

Sensual Body or Room Spray

10 drops jasmine essential oil
10 drops orange essential oil
10 drops rose essential oil

Follow the method for making body sprays, page 29. Combine all the ingredients in a 4-ounce glass bottle, then add enough water to fill the bottle. Put on the spray cap and shake well.

Sexy Sandalwood Blend

2 drops sandalwood essential oil
1 drop rose essential oil
1 drop sweet orange essential oil

Follow the method for making blended oils, page 29. Use per the diffuser manufacturer's instructions.

Variation: For an even sexier spray, use 1 drop jasmine essential oil in place of the sweet orange essential oil.

Spicy Room Spray

1 ounce vodka
20 drops sweet orange essential oil
10 drops black pepper essential oil
10 drops ginger essential oil

Follow the method for making room sprays, page 29. Combine all the ingredients in a 4-ounce glass bottle, then add enough water to fill the bottle. Put on the spray cap and shake well.

ACKNOWLEDGMENTS

I dedicate this book to Henry T. Asselin, an amazing grandfather, storyteller, computer scientist, restaurant owner, rocket man, and friend to all who met him. He never doubted my ability, always had a kind word, and loved my lavender salve. He praised the healing qualities of everything I made, and he made me feel so proud, from the beginning. His joy and belief are something I have the honor of carrying with me every day.

I also must thank Patricia Martin. In the fourth grade, I was friends with her daughter, and she introduced me to essential oils and aromatherapy. Without her, I'm not sure if my interest in aromatherapy would have developed so early and progressed so rapidly. If I had not had this introduction in grade school, I know I would have eventually fallen in love with essential oils, but it would not have happened so early in my life.

I would also like to thank my husband and children for all their support and love.

ABOUT THE AUTHOR

Demetria Clark is an internationally acclaimed herbalist and aromatherapist. In 1998 she advanced online herbal education by founding the first online herbal school, HeartofHerbs.com, which offers herbal and aromatherapy certification programs. Demetria is also a lay midwife and doula and the global director of Birth Arts International. She is a member of the Northeast Herbal Association and the American Herbalists Guild. Demetria received her aromatherapy education from the Pacific Institute of Aromatherapy and the renowned herbal pioneer Jeanne Rose.

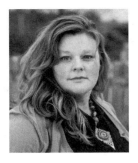

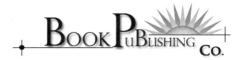

BOOK PUBLISHING CO.

books that educate, inspire, and empower

A Holistic Approach to **ADHD** – *Deborah Merlin*

Weight Loss and Good Health with **APPLE CIDER VINEGAR** – *Cynthia Holzapfel*

Healthy and Beautiful with **COCONUT OIL** – *Cynthia Holzapfel and Laura Holzapfel*

The Weekend **DETOX** – *Jerry Lee Hutchens*

Enhance Your Health with **FERMENTED FOODS** – *Warren Jefferson*

Improve Digestion with **FOOD COMBINING** – *Steve Meyerowitz*

Understanding **GOUT** – *Warren Jefferson*

GREEN SMOOTHIES The Easy Way to Get Your Greens – *Jennifer Cornbleet*

KALE: The Nutritional Powerhouse – *Beverly Lynn Bennett*

PALEO Smoothies – *Alan Roettinger*

Refreshing Fruit and Vegetable **SMOOTHIES** – *Robert Oser*

All titles in the **Live Healthy Now** series are only **$5.95!**

Interested in other health topics or healthy cookbooks?
See our complete line of titles at bookpubco.com or order
directly from:

Book Publishing Company
PO Box 99
Summertown, TN 38483
1-888-260-8458